About the NCCN Guidelines for Patients®

National Comprehensive Cancer Network®

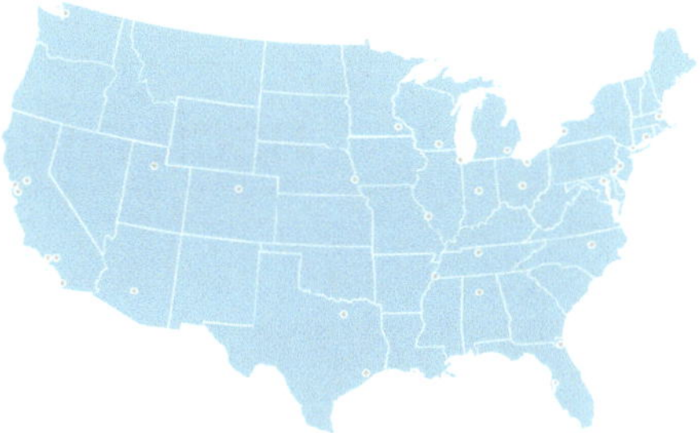

Did you know that top cancer centers across the United States work together to improve cancer care? This alliance of leading cancer centers is called the National Comprehensive Cancer Network® (NCCN®).

Cancer care is always changing. NCCN develops evidence-based cancer care recommendations used by health care providers worldwide. These frequently updated recommendations are the NCCN Clinical Practice Guidelines in Oncology (NCCN Guidelines®). The NCCN Guidelines for Patients plainly explain these expert recommendations for people with cancer and caregivers.

These NCCN Guidelines for Patients are based on the NCCN Clinical Practice Guidelines in Oncology (NCCN Guidelines®) for Chronic Myeloid Leukemia, Version 1.2025 – August 8, 2024.

View the NCCN Guidelines for Patients free online
NCCN.org/patientguidelines

Find an NCCN Cancer Center near you
NCCN.org/cancercenters

Connect with us

Supporters

NCCN Guidelines for Patients are supported by funding from the NCCN Foundation®

NCCN Foundation gratefully acknowledges the following corporate supporters for helping to make available these NCCN Guidelines for Patients: Novartis Pharmaceuticals Corporation and Pfizer Inc.

NCCN independently adapts, updates, and hosts the NCCN Guidelines for Patients. Our corporate supporters do not participate in the development of the NCCN Guidelines for Patients and are not responsible for the content and recommendations contained therein.

To make a gift or learn more, visit online or email

NCCNFoundation.org/donate

PatientGuidelines@NCCN.org

Contents

NCCN Foundation seeks to support the millions of patients and their families affected by a cancer diagnosis by funding and distributing NCCN Guidelines for Patients. NCCN Foundation is also committed to advancing cancer treatment by funding the nation's promising doctors at the center of innovation in cancer research. For more details and the full library of patient and caregiver resources, visit NCCN.org/patients.

National Comprehensive Cancer Network (NCCN) and NCCN Foundation
3025 Chemical Road, Suite 100, Plymouth Meeting, PA 19462 USA

1 About CML

Chronic myeloid leukemia (CML) is caused by a single, specific abnormal gene that is created when a piece of chromosome 9 and a piece of chromosome 22 break off and trade places. The result is a fused gene called *BCR::ABL1* and a shortened chromosome 22 called the Philadelphia (Ph) chromosome. If you do not have the Ph chromosome or the *BCR::ABL1* gene, you do not have CML.

Why you should read this book

Making decisions about cancer care can be stressful. You may need to make tough decisions under pressure about complex choices.

NCCN Guidelines for Patients are trusted by patients and providers. They clearly explain current care recommendations made by respected experts in the field. Recommendations are based on the latest research and practices at leading cancer centers.

Cancer care is not the same for everyone. By following expert recommendations for your situation, you are more likely to improve your care and have better outcomes as a result. Use this book as your guide to find the information you need to make important decisions.

What is CML?

Chronic myeloid leukemia (CML) is a type of blood cancer. Blood is a tissue. A tissue is a group of cells that work together to perform a function. Blood's function is to move oxygen and nutrients throughout your body and carry away waste. Blood also plays an important role for the immune system and in preventing bleeding. There are 4 main components of blood—plasma, red blood cells, white blood cells, and platelets.

Types of blood cells

Your blood contains different types of cells that float in plasma. Plasma is a clear, yellowish fluid made up of mostly water.

There are 3 types of blood cells:

- Red blood cells (RBCs or erythrocytes) carry oxygen throughout the body.
- White blood cells (WBCs or leukocytes), which include granulocytes, monocytes, and lymphocytes, fight infections.
- Platelets (PLTs or thrombocytes) help control bleeding.

In CML, there are usually too many white blood cells (granulocytes). Sometimes, there are too few or too many platelets, as well. Chronic means this cancer worsens slowly.

Granulocytes include:

- Neutrophils
- Eosinophils
- Basophils

How are blood cells formed?

Bone marrow is the sponge-like tissue in the center of most bones. Inside your bone marrow are early blood-forming cells called blood (hematopoietic) stem cells. All types of blood cells are created from blood stem cells. At any given time, the bone marrow will have cells in various stages of development, from very young (immature) to almost fully mature. This process is called differentiation. Blood stem cells give rise to red blood cells (RBCs), white blood cells (WBCs), and platelets (PLTs), which are then released into your bloodstream as needed.

The role of blood stem cells is to make cells called intermediaries that will become red blood cells, white blood cells, and platelets. These intermediaries are called progenitor cells or precursor cells.

There are different types of progenitor cells:

- **Lymphoid progenitor cells** form into lymphoblasts that mature into lymphocytes.

Philadelphia chromosome

Chronic myeloid leukemia (CML) is caused by a single, specific abnormal gene that is created when a piece of chromosome 9 and a piece of chromosome 22 break off and trade places. The result is a fused gene called *BCR::ABL1* and a shortened chromosome 22 called the Philadelphia (Ph) chromosome.

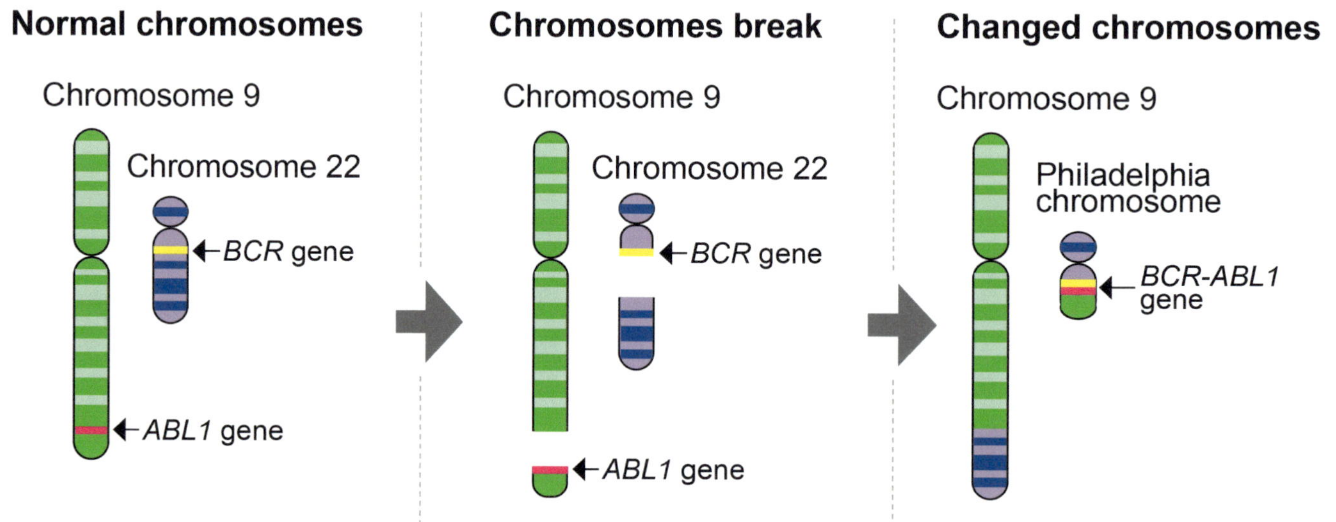

- **Myeloid progenitor cells** form into myeloblasts and other non-lymphoid blood cells.

Often, in CML the very immature or most immature cells (myeloblasts or lymphoblasts) are referred to simply as blasts.

CML is thought to arise from blood stem cells that make an increased amount of myeloid progenitor cells. However, an advanced form of CML, called blast phase CML (BP-CML), can cause an increased amount of lymphoid or myeloid progenitor cells. The type of blast phase cell will affect treatment in BP-CML.

What causes CML?

The cause of CML can be traced to a single, specific abnormal gene called *BCR::ABL1*. This fused gene occurs when a piece of chromosome 9 and a piece of chromosome 22 break off and switch places. This creates a new, abnormal chromosome 22 that contains a small part of chromosome 9. This new chromosome is referred to as the Philadelphia chromosome (Ph) and is the hallmark of CML. If you do not have the Ph chromosome or the *BCR::ABL1* gene, you do not have CML. *BCR::ABL1* is not found in normal blood cells. It is not passed down from birth parents to children. The *BCR::ABL1* gene makes a new protein that leads to uncontrolled blood cell growth. This growth ultimately leads to CML. Treatment for CML aims to stop the activity of the BCR::ABL1 protein.

Those with CML should be treated at centers experienced in this type of cancer.

What can you do to get the best care?

Advocate for yourself. You have an important role to play in your care. In fact, you're more likely to get the care you want by asking questions and making shared decisions with your care team. Consider seeking the opinion of a CML specialist.

The *NCCN Guidelines for Patients* will help you understand cancer care. With better understanding, you'll be more prepared to discuss your care with your team and share your concerns. Many people feel more satisfied when they play an active role in their care.

You may not know what to ask your care team. That's common. Each chapter in this book ends with an important section called *Questions to ask*. These suggested questions will help you get more information on all aspects of your care.

Take the next step and keep reading to learn what is the best care for you!

This book is organized into chapters on:

- Testing
- Treatment
- CML phases

2
Tests

Treatment planning starts with testing. Accurate testing is needed to diagnose and treat CML. This chapter presents an overview of possible tests you might receive and what to expect.

Test results

Results from blood tests and possible biopsy will be used to determine your treatment plan. Treatment will be based on these findings.

It is important you understand what these tests mean. Ask questions about your test results. Online patient portals are one way to access your test results.

Keep these things in mind:

- It's beneficial to have a support system in place during diagnosis and treatment. Enlist the help of friends, family members, or peers who can provide transportation, meals, and emotional support. These can be different people for different tasks or change over time.
- Consider bringing someone with you to doctor visits if possible, or have someone on the phone or join you for telehealth visits.
- Don't hesitate to ask questions and take notes during appointments. Write down questions and ask a friend or family member to take notes. Caregivers should ask questions, too.
- Organize your medical documents, including insurance forms, medical records, and test results. Keep a list of contact information for your care team and update your primary care physician (PCP) regarding any changes. Include details about the specific type of cancer, treatment, and dates on your contact list.
- Ask your care team how best to communicate with them, especially in an emergency.

Tests used to diagnose CML can be found in **Guide 1.**

Guide 1 Testing for CML
Medical history and physical exam that includes spleen size
Complete blood count (CBC) with differential
Chemistry profile, including uric acid
Bone marrow aspirate and biopsy
qPCR using IS for *BCR::ABL1* found in blood
Hepatitis B panel

General health tests

Some general health tests are described next.

Medical history

A medical history is a record of all health issues and treatments you have had in your life. Be prepared to list any illness or injury and when it happened. Bring a list of old and new medicines and any over-the-counter (OTC) medicines, herbals, or supplements you take. Some supplements interact with and affect medicines that your care team may prescribe. Tell your care team about any symptoms you have. A medical history, sometimes called a health history, will help determine which treatment is best for you.

Family history

To date, there is no compelling evidence that having a family history of CML increases the chances of developing CML. However, other cancers and diseases can run in families. Your care team will ask about the health history of family members who are blood relatives. This information is called a family history. Ask family members on both sides of your family about their health issues like heart disease, cancer, and diabetes, and at what age they were diagnosed. It's important to know the specific type of cancer or where the cancer started, if it is in multiple locations, and if they had genetic testing.

Physical exam

During a physical exam, your health care provider may:

- Check your temperature, blood pressure, pulse, and breathing rate
- Check your height and weight
- Listen to your lungs and heart
- Look in your eyes, ears, nose, and throat
- Feel and apply pressure to parts of your body to see if organs are of normal size, are soft or hard, or cause pain when touched
- Feel for enlarged lymph nodes in your neck, underarm, and groin
- Feel your abdomen and below your left ribcage to see if your spleen is enlarged. An enlarged spleen is one sign of CML.

Blood tests

Blood tests check for signs of disease and how well organs are working. They require a sample of your blood, which is removed through a needle placed into a vein in your arm. Some blood tests are described next.

Blood clotting tests

Your body stops bleeding by turning blood into a gel-like form. The gel-like blood forms into a solid mass called a blood clot. Clotting is a process or series of events. Proteins, called coagulation factors, are needed for clotting. They are made by the liver. These tests are known together as a coagulation panel or disseminated intravascular coagulation (DIC) panel.

An impaired clotting process is common in leukemia. This is called coagulopathy. You may have bleeding and bruises or blood clots.

Complete blood count and differential

A complete blood count (CBC) measures the levels of red blood cells (RBCs), white blood cells (WBCs), and platelets (PLTs) in your blood. A CBC is a key test that gives a picture of your overall bone marrow health. A differential counts the number of each type of WBC (neutrophils, lymphocytes, monocytes, eosinophils, and basophils). It also checks if the counts are in balance with each other. CML often causes a high WBC count and/or high PLT count but can sometimes cause low RBC counts.

Chemistry profile

A chemistry profile or panel measures the levels of different substances released into your blood by the liver, bone, and other organs.

Creatinine

Creatinine is a waste produced in the muscles. Every person generates a fixed amount of creatinine every day based on how much muscle they have. It is filtered out of the blood by the kidneys. The level of creatinine in the blood tells how well the kidneys are working. Higher levels of creatinine mean the kidneys aren't working as well as when someone had lower levels of creatinine.

Be prepared to have many blood tests.

Hepatitis B panel

Hepatitis is a virus that causes inflammation of the liver. Hepatitis B virus (HBV) is spread by contact with blood and other bodily fluids. A blood test will show if you had hepatitis in the past or if you have it today. Some treatments might cause HBV to reactivate, which can cause liver damage. There are ways to prevent or treat reactivation.

HLA typing

Human leukocyte antigen (HLA) is a protein found on the surface of most cells. It plays an important role in your body's immune response. HLAs are unique to each person. They mark your body's cells. Your body detects these markers to tell which cells are yours. In other words, all your cells have the same set of HLAs. Each person's set of HLAs is called the HLA type or tissue type.

HLA typing is a blood test that detects a person's HLA type. This test is done before a donor (allogeneic) hematopoietic cell transplant. To find a donor match, your proteins will be compared to the donor's white blood cells to see how many proteins are the same. A very good match is needed for a transplant to be a treatment option. Otherwise, your body will reject the donor cells or the donor cells will react against your body. Blood samples from you and your blood relatives will be tested first.

Liver function tests

Liver function tests (LFTs) look at the health of your liver by measuring chemicals that are made or processed by the liver. Levels that are too high or low signal that the liver is not working well.

Pregnancy test

Those who can become pregnant will be given a pregnancy test before treatment begins.

Uric acid

Uric acid is released by cells when DNA breaks down. It is a normal waste product that dissolves in the blood and is filtered by the kidneys where it leaves the body in the urine. Too much uric acid in the body is called hyperuricemia. With CML, it can be caused by fast turnover (cell death) of white blood cells (WBCs). High uric acid might be a side effect of treatment. Very high levels of uric acid in the blood can cause kidney stones, kidney damage, and gout (inflammation of joints). You may be prescribed allopurinol for a brief period of time after starting primary treatment.

Fertility (all genders)

Treatment with targeted therapy and other forms of systemic therapy can affect your fertility, or the ability to have children. If you think you want children in the future, ask your care team how cancer and cancer treatment might affect your fertility.

Fertility preservation is all about keeping your options open, whether you know you want to have children later in life or aren't sure at the moment. Fertility and reproductive specialists can help you sort through what may be best for your situation.

More information on fertility preservation can be found at NCCN.org/patientguidelines and on the NCCN Patient Guides for Cancer app.

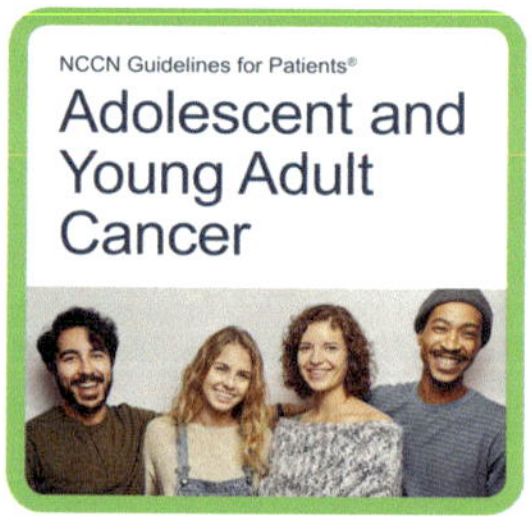

Performance status

Performance status (PS) is a person's general level of fitness and ability to perform daily tasks. Your state of general health will be rated using a PS scale called the Eastern Cooperative Oncology Group (ECOG) score or the Karnofsky Performance Status (KPS). PS is one factor taken into consideration when choosing a treatment plan. Your preferences about treatment are always important.

Bone marrow tests

Leukemia starts in the bone marrow. To diagnose CML and determine the CML phase, samples of bone marrow are collected and tested before starting any treatment. Although this can sometimes be a painful procedure, your care team will try to make you as comfortable as possible. Usually, you will only have this test once at diagnosis. However, you might have it again during or after treatment, if needed.

There are 2 types of bone marrow tests that are often done at the same time:

- Bone marrow aspirate
- Bone marrow biopsy

Samples of bone and marrow are removed in a bone marrow biopsy. A bone marrow aspirate and biopsy is needed to diagnose CML.

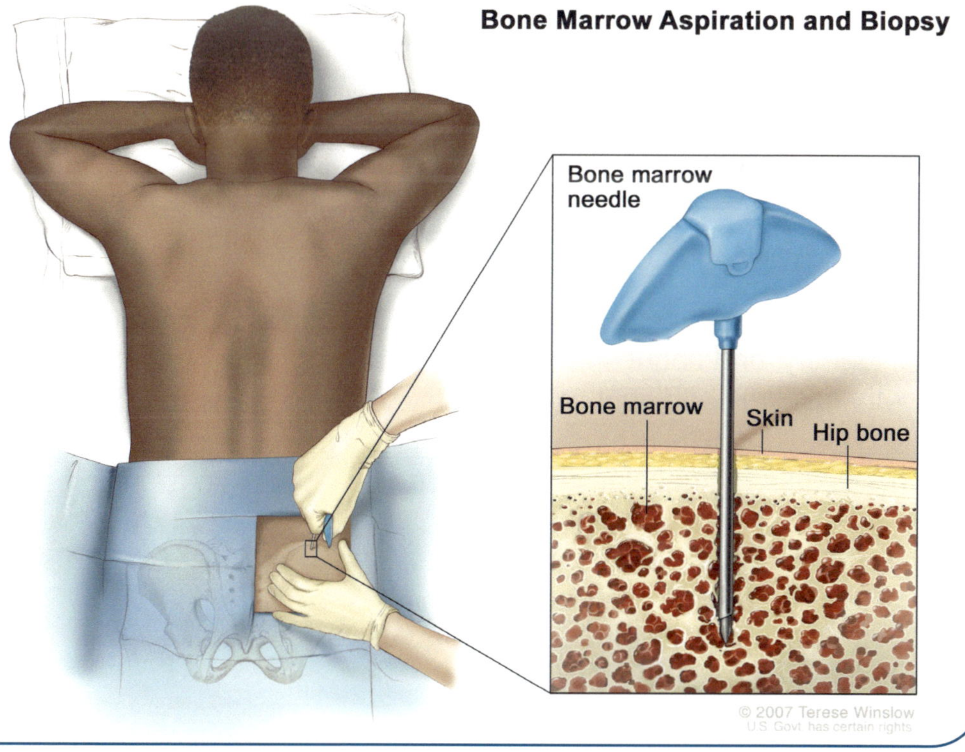

Your bone marrow is like a sponge holding liquid and cells. An aspirate takes some of the liquid and cells out of the sponge, and a biopsy takes a piece of the sponge.

The samples are usually taken from the back of the hip bone (pelvis). You will likely lie on your belly or side. Your doctors will first clean your skin, then give sedation and/or numb your skin and outer surface of your bone. For an aspirate, a hollow needle will be pushed through your skin and into the bone. Liquid bone marrow will then be drawn into a syringe. For the biopsy, a wider needle will be used to remove a core sample. You may feel bone pain at your hip for a few days. Your skin may bruise.

Your bone marrow sample should be reviewed by a pathologist who is an expert in the diagnosis of CML. This review is often referred to as histology, histopathology, or hematopathology review. The pathologist will note the overall appearance and the size, shape, and type of your cells. Tests will be done on the biopsied cells. Ask questions about your biopsy results and what it means for your treatment.

Flow cytometry

Flow cytometry is a laboratory method used to detect, identify, and count specific cells. Flow cytometry involves adding a light-sensitive dye to cells. The dyed cells are passed through a beam of light in a machine. The machine measures the number of cells.

Flow cytometry may be used on cells from circulating (peripheral) blood or from a bone marrow aspirate. A blood test can count the number of white blood cells (WBCs), but it cannot detect the subtle differences between different types of blood cancers. Flow cytometry can help detect these subtle differences.

Testing for CML biomarker and genetic changes

Biomarker and genetic tests are used to learn more about your type of CML, to target treatment, and to determine the likely path your cancer will take (prognosis). This genetic testing is different from family history genetic testing or genetic cancer risk testing. This testing looks for changes only in the CML cells that have developed over time, and not changes in the rest of your body's cells. Testing will look for the Philadelphia (Ph) chromosome, which is used to diagnose and to help determine the CML phase. You may be placed into a risk group based on the types of genetic abnormalities found.

Inside our cells are DNA (deoxyribonucleic acid) molecules. These molecules are tightly packaged into what is called a chromosome. Chromosomes contain most of the genetic information in a cell. Normal human cells contain 23 pairs of chromosomes for a total of 46 chromosomes. Each chromosome contains thousands of genes. Genes are coded instructions for the proteins your cells make. A mutation is when something goes wrong in the genetic code. Proteins are written like this: BCR::ABL1. Genes are written in italics like this: *BCR::ABL1*.

Mutation testing

Mutation testing uses methods such as karyotype, fluorescence in situ hybridization (FISH), polymerase chain reaction (PCR), and next-generation sequencing (NGS) to look for changes or abnormalities that are unique to CML cells (genes and chromosomes). Some mutations may determine the type of treatment given. Subtle new drug-resistant mutations in the *BCR::ABL1* gene may emerge over time. They can happen as CML progresses to advanced phases such as accelerated or blast phase. Some mutations lead to resistance to certain targeted therapies. There are many possible mutations.

FISH

Fluorescence in situ hybridization (FISH) is a method that involves special dyes called probes that attach to pieces of DNA. For example, the probes attach to the *BCR* gene and the *ABL1* gene. The *BCR::ABL1* gene is detected when the colors of the probes overlap by translocation. A translocation is the switching of parts between two chromosomes. The *BCR::ABL1* translocation can also be written as t(9;22).

FISH can look for translocations that are too small to be seen with other methods. It can only be used for known changes. It cannot detect all the possible changes found within genes or chromosomes. A bone marrow sample is often needed to get all the information your care team needs to plan your care.

Karyotype

A karyotype is a picture of your chromosomes. The study of chromosomes is called cytogenetics.

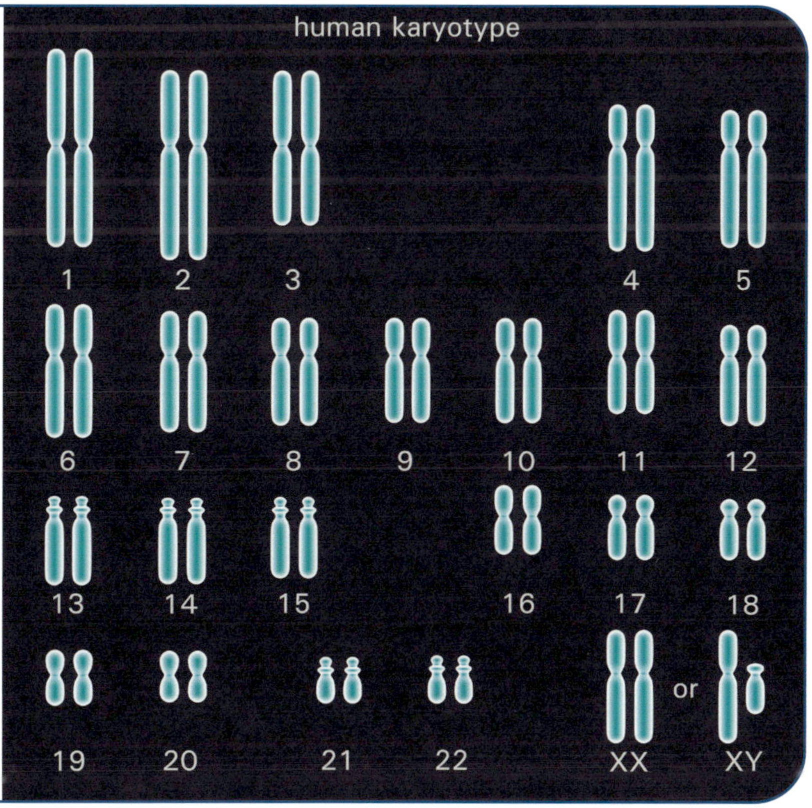

Karyotype

A karyotype is a picture of chromosomes. Normal human cells contain 23 pairs of chromosomes for a total of 46 chromosomes. A karyotype will show extra, missing, rearranged, or abnormal pieces of chromosomes. Since a karyotype requires growing cells, a sample of bone marrow or blood must be used.

Chromosome translocation and gene rearrangement

Chromosome translocation and gene rearrangement is the switching of parts between 2 chromosomes. When described at the chromosome level, it is called a translocation. When described at the gene level, it is called rearrangement. For example, a translocation between chromosome 9 and 22 is written as t(9;22) and is known as the Philadelphia (Ph) chromosome. Its gene rearrangement is written as *BCR::ABL1*.

Next-generation sequencing

Next-generation sequencing (NGS) is a method used to determine a portion of a person's DNA sequence. It shows if a gene has any mutations that might affect how the gene works. NGS looks at the gene in a more detailed way than other methods and can find mutations that other methods might miss.

PCR

A polymerase chain reaction (PCR) is a technique that can make millions or billions of copies of your DNA or RNA (genetic information). PCR is very sensitive. It can find 1 abnormal cell among more than 100,000 normal cells. These copies, called PCR products, might be used for NGS.

qPCR (IS)

A special PCR called quantitative reverse transcriptase polymerase chain reaction (qPCR) is used in CML. It measures the proportion of cells with the *BCR::ABL1* gene compared to normal cells with a gene needed for maintaining basic cell functions (called a housekeeping gene) such as *ABL1.* The number found in your blood is compared to an international standard or baseline called the International Scale (IS). This is the most important test for monitoring response to treatment. Ask your care team if they are using qPCR (IS). It is the gold standard for detecting and measuring *BCR::ABL1*.

A qPCR (IS) should be done at initial diagnosis to look for the presence of the *BCR::ABL1* gene on the Philadelphia chromosome. You will have this test often after starting treatment. This test might be referred to as real-time or reverse transcriptase (RT)-PCR. The qPCR level of *BCR::ABL1* shows how your disease is responding to CML therapy and is an important measure of your progress.

Heart tests

Heart or cardiac tests are used to see how well your heart works. These tests might be used to monitor treatment side effects. You might be referred to a cardiologist.

Electrocardiogram

An electrocardiogram (ECG or EKG) shows electrical changes in your heart. It reveals information about your heart rate and rhythm. A prolonged corrected QT interval (or QTc) occurs when your heart muscle takes longer than normal to recharge between beats. Often, this electrical disturbance can be seen on an ECG. Certain treatments for CML can cause a prolonged QTc. If the QTc becomes too prolonged, it can cause dangerous heart rhythms.

Echocardiogram

An echocardiogram (or echo) uses sound waves to make pictures. It is a type of ultrasound. For this test, small patches will be placed on your chest to track your heartbeat. Next, a wand with gel on its tip will be slid across part of your bare chest. A picture of your beating heart will be seen on a screen. The pictures will be recorded for future viewing.

An echocardiogram is one way of measuring ejection fraction, which is the amount of blood pumped out of the left side of your heart every time it beats. In low ejection fraction, the amount of blood pumping from the left side of the heart is lower than normal.

Seek out support groups at your local hospital, through social media, or through resources listed in the back of this book. Look to friends, relatives, neighbors, and coworkers for social support.

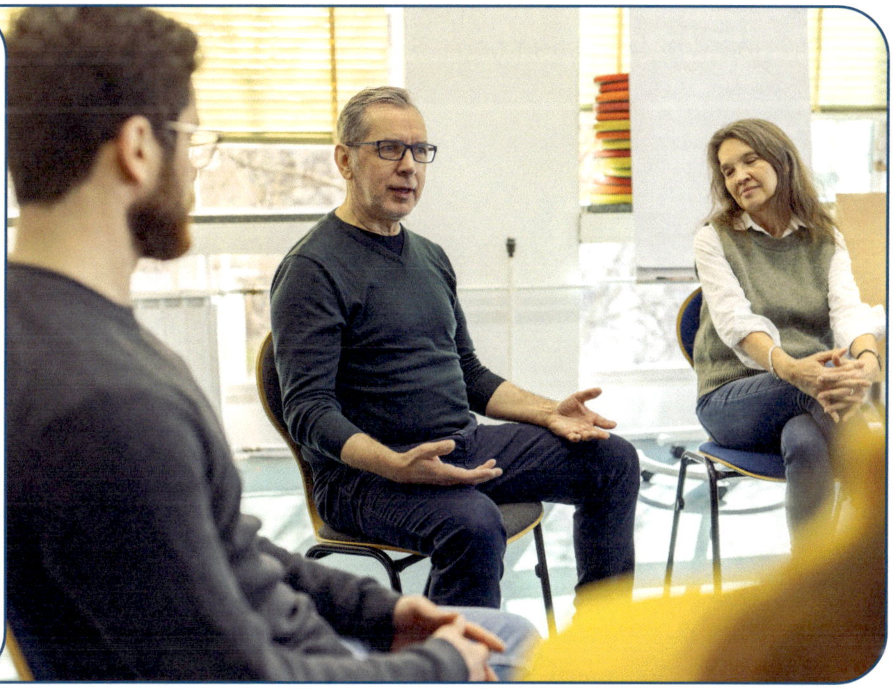

Key points

- A diagnosis of chronic myeloid leukemia (CML) is confirmed using a bone marrow aspirate and bone marrow biopsy.
- Genetic and biomarker tests are used to learn more about your CML, to target treatment, and to determine the likely course your cancer will take called a prognosis.
- A special polymerase chain reaction (PCR) called quantitative reverse transcriptase PCR (qPCR) using the International Scale (IS) measures the proportion of cells with the *BCR::ABL1* gene mutation.
- In some cases, CML cells can develop additional mutations, which can affect treatment options. Therefore, you might have mutation testing before treatment for advanced phase CML.
- Talk to your care team if you are or plan to become pregnant. Certain treatments for CML will need to be avoided if you are pregnant or breastfeeding.

Questions to ask

- What type of cancer do I have? What does this mean in terms of my prognosis and treatment options?
- Is there a cancer center or hospital nearby that specializes in this type of cancer?
- What tests will I have? How often will they be repeated?
- Will my insurance pay for this test?
- Who will talk with me about the next steps and when?

3
Treating CML

This chapter presents an overview of therapies you might receive. CML is usually treated with targeted therapy. A targeted therapy focuses on specific or unique features of cancer cells such as the protein made by the *BCR::ABL1* gene.

Chronic myeloid leukemia (CML) is highly treatable and may be curable in certain circumstances. It is important to have regular talks with your care team about your goals for treatment and your treatment plan.

Care team

Treating CML takes a team approach. Treatment decisions should involve a multidisciplinary team (MDT). An MDT is a team of health care and psychosocial care professionals from different professional backgrounds who have knowledge (expertise) and experience in your type of cancer. This team is united in the planning and implementing of your treatment. Ask who will coordinate your care.

Some members of your care team will be with you throughout cancer treatment, while others will only be there for parts of it. Get to know your care team and help them get to know you.

You know your body better than anyone

Help your care team understand:

- How you feel
- What you need
- What is working and what is not

Keep a list of names and contact information for each member of your team. This will make it easier for you and anyone involved in your care to know whom to contact with questions or concerns.

Get to know your care team and help them get to know you.

Your team might include the following specialists:

- **A hematologist or hematologic oncologist** is a medical expert in blood diseases and blood cancers.
- **A medical oncologist** treats cancer in adults using systemic (drug) therapy.
- **A pathologist or hematopathologist** analyzes the cells and tissues removed during a biopsy and provides cancer diagnosis, staging, and information about biomarker testing.

Three phases of CML

CML can have three phases. Most people with CML are diagnosed in the chronic phase, but a small number can be diagnosed in the accelerated or blast phase. Some people with CML progress from chronic phase to accelerated or blast phase.

The 3 phases of CML are:

- Chronic
- Accelerated
- Blast

Phases are based on the percentage of immature white blood cells (blasts) found in the blood and bone marrow. Normal bone marrow contains up to 5 percent (5%) blasts. This means that it is normal to have less than 5 blasts for every 100 blood cells. In CML the number of blasts may be higher than 5%, but is usually less than 15%. Fifteen percent or more blasts is a sign of advanced phase CML. Accelerated and blast phase are considered advanced phases.

Chronic phase

The first phase of CML is called chronic phase (CP-CML). In this phase, there is an increased number of white blood cells in the blood, bone marrow, or both. Less than 15 out of every 100 blood cells are myeloblasts (<15%).

CML typically progresses very slowly in the chronic phase. It may take several months or years to reach the next phase. Compared to other phases, CP-CML typically responds better to treatment.

Accelerated phase

The second phase of CML is called accelerated phase (AP-CML). In this phase, the number of myeloblasts is higher than normal or there are chromosome changes that suggest that the number of myeloblasts is going to increase soon. The number of white blood cells may also be high. Other cells called promyelocytes and eosinophils may be increased. There may be a very low number of platelets in the blood caused by CML and not by treatment. In the accelerated phase, CML cells may grow faster.

In all phases, CML cells contain the Philadelphia chromosome (Ph+). However, in the accelerated phase, there may be new abnormal DNA changes (mutations) within Ph+ cells.

Blast phase

The third and final phase of CML is called blast phase (BP-CML) or blast crisis. Once CML is in blast phase, it can be life-threatening and very difficult to treat. As a result, a major focus of treatment of CML is to prevent blast phase. Blast phase happens after a series of events, including additional gene mutations and resistance to targeted drug therapy. However, some people are first diagnosed as having BP-CML (before any treatment).

A blast is a very immature white blood cell. There is more than one type of white blood cell. Both lymphoid and myeloid progenitor cells form into blast cells called lymphoblasts or myeloblasts depending on the type. Blasts are committed to becoming a type of blood cell. Lymphoblasts normally mature into lymphocytes, a type of white blood cell. Myeloblasts are responsible for all other non-lymphoid blood cells in bone marrow, such as granulocytes, a type of white blood cell, as well as platelets. However, in the blast phase of CML, the normal maturation process is impaired.

- **In myeloid BP-CML,** the number of myeloblasts is very high, at least 30 out of every 100 cells (30%).
- **In lymphoid BP-CML,** any number of abnormal lymphoblasts is concerning.

Blast cells may be found in tissues and organs outside the bone marrow or blood. Treatment for BP-CML is based on whether the blasts are myeloid or lymphoid.

Systemic therapy

CML is treated with systemic therapy. Systemic therapy is drug therapy that works throughout the body. It includes targeted therapy, immunotherapy, and chemotherapy. CML is usually treated with targeted therapy. Goals of systemic therapy should be discussed before starting treatment. The choice of therapy takes into consideration many factors, including age, other serious health issues, and future treatment possibilities like a hematopoietic cell transplant (HCT). Your preferences about treatment are important. If you have any religious or personal beliefs about certain kinds of treatment, now would be the time to share them with your care team.

Chemotherapy

Chemotherapy kills fast-dividing cells throughout the body, including cancer cells and normal cells.

Standard of care is the best-known way to treat a particular disease based on past clinical trials. There may be more than one treatment regimen that is considered standard of care. Ask your care team what treatment options are available and if a clinical trial might be right for you.

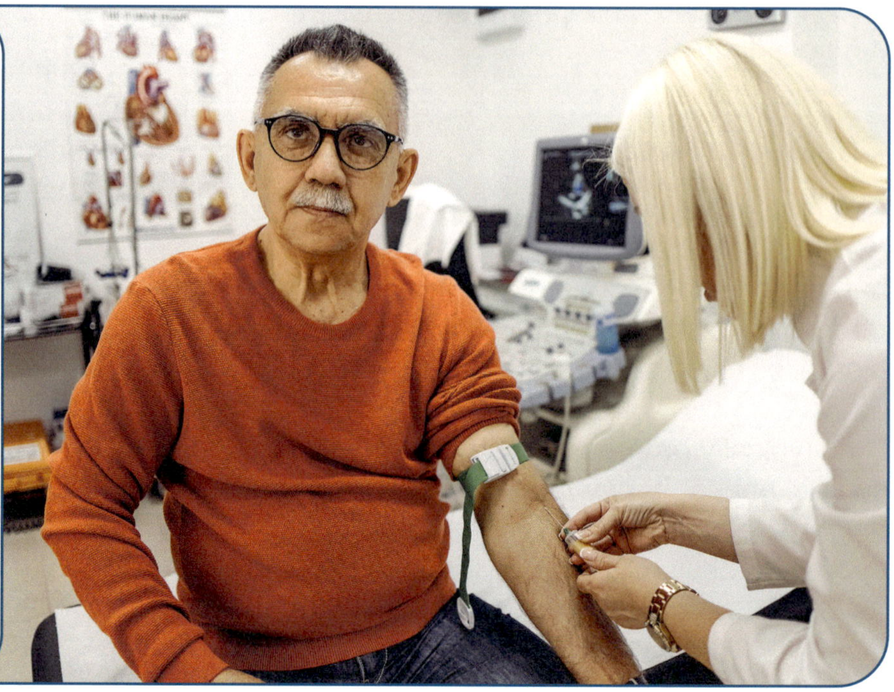

Steroids

Steroid is the short name for corticosteroid. Steroids are man-made versions of hormones made by the adrenal glands. The adrenal glands are small structures found near the kidneys, which help regulate blood pressure and reduce inflammation. Steroids also are toxic to lymphoid cells and may be part of a treatment. Steroids can cause short-term and long-term side effects.

Targeted therapy

Targeted therapy is a form of systemic therapy that focuses on specific or unique features of cancer cells. Targeted therapies seek out how cancer cells grow, divide, and move in the body. These drugs stop the action of molecules that help cancer cells grow and/or survive.

Tyrosine kinase inhibitor

A tyrosine kinase inhibitor (TKI) is a type of targeted therapy that blocks the signals that cause cancer to grow and spread. TKIs might be used alone or in combination with other systemic therapies like chemotherapy and immunotherapy.

Tyrosine kinases are proteins in cells that are important for many cell functions. The protein made by the *BCR::ABL1* gene is a tyrosine kinase. It moves or transfers chemicals, called phosphates, from one molecule to another. TKIs block this transfer, which stops the uncontrolled cell growth in CML.

TKIs are slightly different from one another, but they generally work in a similar way. They may cause different side effects. You might

Warnings about supplements and drug interactions

You might be asked to stop taking or avoid certain herbal supplements when on a systemic therapy. Some supplements can affect the ability of a drug to do its job. This is called a drug interaction.

It is critical to speak with your care team about any supplements you may be taking. Some examples include:

- Turmeric
- Ginkgo biloba
- Green tea extract
- St. John's Wort
- Antioxidants

Certain medicines can also affect the ability of a drug to do its job. Antacids, heart or blood pressure medicine, and antidepressants are just some of the medicines that might interact with a systemic therapy or supportive care medicines given during systemic therapy. Therefore, it is very important to tell your care team about any medicines, vitamins, over-the-counter (OTC) drugs, herbals, or supplements you are taking.

Bring a list with you to every visit.

not be given a certain TKI if you have a health condition, such as lung or heart issues, or certain mutations. Sometimes, a TKI will stop working if there's a new drug-resistant mutation in CML cells. Switching to a different TKI can often help.

TKIs used to treat CML

TKIs that might be used to treat CML (listed in alphabetical order):

- Asciminib (Scemblix)
- Bosutinib (Bosulif)
- Dasatinib (Sprycel)
- Imatinib (Gleevec)
- Nilotinib (Tasigna)
- Ponatinib (Iclusig)

TKIs are divided into first, second, and even third generation. In general, each generation of a drug gets more specific and better at targeting certain mutations. This means that second- and third-generation TKIs are usually more specific, more potent, and better at targeting certain mutations. However, they might have more side effects. TKI options will be based on your specific situation.

If CML doesn't seem to be responding to one TKI, then another TKI will be tried. Certain drugs may work better and be less toxic. Dose might be increased or decreased depending on how CML is responding to treatment. You will be closely monitored during treatment.

Breastfeeding

Those on TKI therapy should not breastfeed. TKIs can pass into human breast milk. If you are breastfeeding or plan to breastfeed, talk to your care team. There are options.

TKI side effects

TKIs can cause side effects. If you feel unwell or a side effect is interfering with your ability to do daily tasks, tell your care team. There may be ways to help you feel better. It is very important to continue to take your medicine even if you do not feel well. Speak to your care team before making any changes!

Side effects are common among TKIs. These include low blood counts, fatigue, and musculoskeletal pain. You may feel nauseated, have diarrhea, and vomit. Changes in your skin may occur, such as a rash. You may feel tired and get headaches and fevers. Fluid buildup in limbs (edema) or around certain organs may occur. Severe side effects include heart and liver issues, and kidney failure. Do not take TKIs while pregnant or breastfeeding. Talk to your care team first before stopping any TKI.

Asciminib

Asciminib is in a separate class because it targets a different area of *BCR::ABL1*. It is a treatment for those with chronic phase CML with a *BCR::ABL1* gene mutation called T315I or may be used as a third-line treatment option in those with chronic phase CML without T315I. It should be avoided in people who have had pancreatitis.

Bosutinib

Bosutinib is a second-generation TKI. It may not be preferred for those who have liver or stomach and digestion (gastrointestinal) issues.

Dasatinib

Dasatinib is a second-generation TKI. It may not be prescribed if you have lung (pulmonary) disease or breathing issues. There is a lower-cost generic dasatinib option.

Imatinib

Imatinib was the first TKI approved by the U.S. FDA (Food and Drug Administration) to treat CML. Imatinib has been studied for a long time and is still a very good treatment option. It is a good option for those who are older, who have other more serious health issues, or for those who have low-risk chronic phase CML where an aggressive treatment might not be needed. There is a lower-cost generic imatinib option.

Nilotinib

Nilotinib is a second-generation TKI. Nilotinib may not be best for those who have heart (cardiovascular) issues, are at risk for heart issues, or who have electrolyte abnormalities. Sudden deaths have occurred in those taking nilotinib. Nilotinib may cause increased blood sugar or worsen peripheral vascular disease. Nilotinib prolongs the QT interval, which is detectable on an electrocardiogram (ECG or EKG). You will likely have ECGs to monitor your heart.

Ponatinib

Ponatinib is a third-generation (3G) TKI. It is the preferred treatment for those with a *BCR::ABL1* gene mutation called T315I, but may be used as a second- or third-line treatment option in those without T315I. Ponatinib can have some serious side effects and is not used as a first-line therapy. You might be referred to a cardiologist to monitor your heart if you receive this treatment.

Your preferences about treatment are always important. If you have any religious or personal beliefs about certain kinds of treatment, share them with your care team and make your wishes known. Together, you and your care team will choose a treatment plan that is best for you.

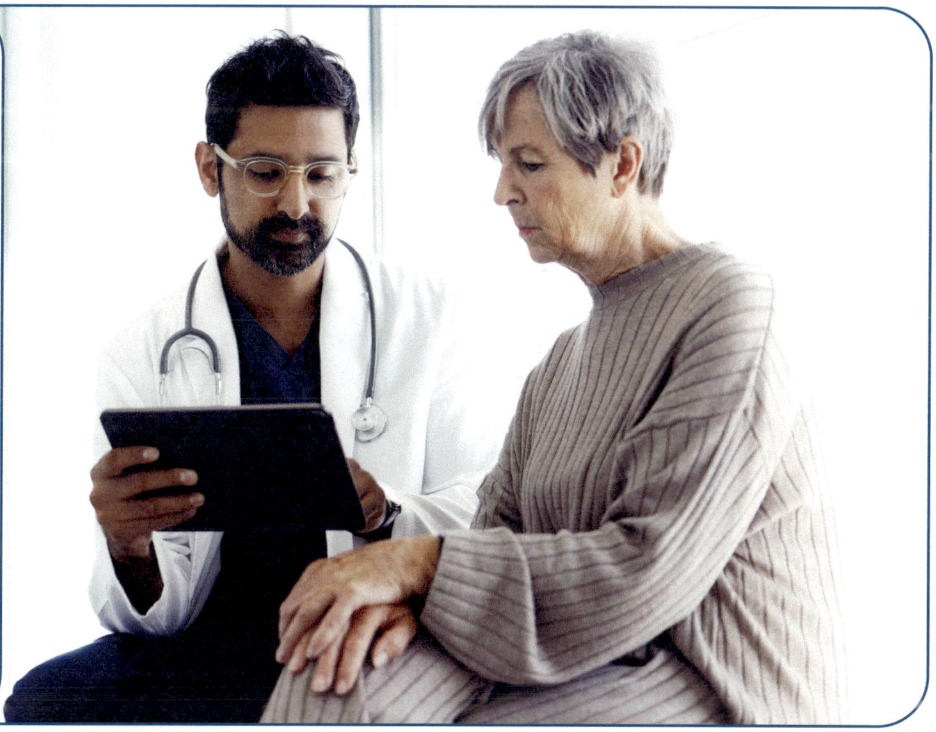

Hematopoietic cell transplant

A hematopoietic cell transplant (HCT) replaces hematopoietic stem cells that have been destroyed by high doses of chemotherapy and/or radiation therapy as part of the transplant process. A hematopoietic stem cell is a very immature cell that can develop into any type of blood cell. You might hear it called a stem cell transplant (SCT) or a bone marrow transplant (BMT). This book will refer to it as HCT. HCTs are performed in specialized centers. Most people with CML do not need an HCT.

There are 2 types of HCTs:

- **Autologous** – stem cells come from you.
- **Allogeneic** – stem cells come from a donor who may or may not be related to you. Only an allogeneic HCT is used as a possible treatment option in CML.

Allogeneic HCT

An allogeneic HCT uses healthy stem cells from a donor. The donor may or may not be related to you. Before an HCT, treatment is needed to destroy bone marrow cells. This is called conditioning and it creates room for the healthy donor stem cells. It also weakens the immune system so your body will accept and won't kill the transplanted cells. Chemotherapy is used for conditioning. Radiation therapy may also be given as part of conditioning treatment.

After conditioning, you will receive a transfusion of the healthy stem cells from a donor that has been matched to you. A transfusion is a slow injection of blood products into a vein. This can take several hours. The transplanted stem cells will travel to your bone marrow and grow. New, healthy blood cells will form. This is called engraftment. It usually takes about 2 to 4 weeks. Until then, you will have little or no immune defense. You may need to stay in a very clean room at the hospital or be given antibiotics to prevent or treat infection. Transfusions are also possible. A red blood cell transfusion is used to prevent bleeding and to treat anemia (below normal red blood cell count). A platelet transfusion is used to treat a low platelet count or bleeding. While waiting for the cells to engraft, you will likely feel tired and weak. This treatment has very serious and life-threatening side effects.

Possible side effects

Every treatment has side effects. You will be monitored for infections, disease relapse, and graft-versus-host disease (GVHD). In GVHD, the donor cells attack your normal, healthy tissue. There are treatments for GVHD. Ask your care team about the possible side effects or complications of HCT and how this might affect your quality of life.

More information on GVHD can be found at NCCN.org/patientguidelines and on the NCCN Patient Guides for Cancer app.

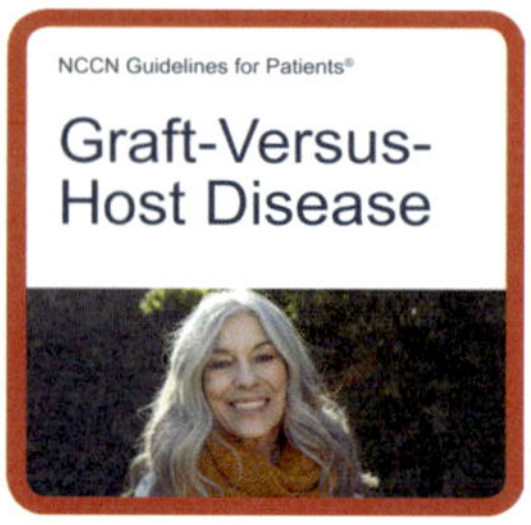

Clinical trials

A clinical trial is a type of medical research study. After being developed and tested in a lab, potential new ways of treating cancer need to be studied in people. If found to be safe and effective in a clinical trial, a drug, device, or treatment approach may be approved by the U.S. Food and Drug Administration (FDA).

Everyone with cancer should carefully consider all of the treatment options available for their cancer type, including standard treatments and clinical trials. Talk to your doctor about whether a clinical trial may make sense for you.

Phases

Most cancer clinical trials focus on treatment and are done in phases.

- **Phase 1** trials study the safety and side effects of an investigational drug or treatment approach.
- **Phase 2** trials study how well the drug or approach works against a specific type of cancer.
- **Phase 3** trials test the drug or approach against a standard treatment. If the results are good, it may be approved by the FDA.
- **Phase 4** trials study the safety and benefit of an FDA-approved treatment.

Who can enroll?

It depends on the clinical trial's rules, called eligibility criteria. The rules may be about age, cancer type and stage, treatment history, or general health. They ensure that participants are alike in specific ways and that the trial is as safe as possible for the participants.

Informed consent

Clinical trials are managed by a research team. This group of experts will review the study with you in detail, including its purpose and the risks and benefits of joining. All of this information is also provided in an informed consent form. Read the form carefully and ask questions before signing it. Take time to discuss it with people you trust. Keep in mind that you can leave and seek treatment outside of the clinical trial at any time.

Will I get a placebo?

Placebos (inactive versions of real medicines) are almost never used alone in cancer clinical trials. It is common to receive either a placebo with a standard treatment, or a new drug with a standard treatment. You will be informed, verbally and in writing, if a placebo is part of a clinical trial before you enroll.

Are clinical trials free?

There is no fee to enroll in a clinical trial. The study sponsor pays for research-related costs, including the study drug. But you may need to pay for other services, like transportation or childcare, due to extra appointments. During the trial, you will continue to receive standard cancer care. This care is often covered by insurance.

General supportive care

Supportive care helps improve your quality of life during and after cancer treatment. The goal is to prevent or manage side effects and symptoms, like pain and cancer-related fatigue. It also addresses the mental, social, and spiritual concerns faced by those with cancer.

Supportive care is available to everyone with cancer and their families, not just those at the end of life. Palliative care is another name for supportive care.

Supportive care can also help with:

- Making treatment decisions
- Coordinating your care
- Paying for care
- Planning for advanced care and end of life

Side effects

All cancer treatments can cause side effects. Side effects depend on many factors. These factors include the drug type and dose, length of treatment, and the person. Some side effects may be harmful to your health. Others may just be unpleasant. Treatment can cause several side effects. Some are very serious.

Ask for a complete list of side effects of your treatments. Also, tell your care team about any new or worsening symptoms. There may be ways to help you feel better. There are also ways to prevent some side effects. You will be monitored closely for side effects.

All cancer treatments can cause unwanted health issues called side effects. It is important to tell your care team about all of your side effects so they can be managed.

Late effects

Late effects are side effects that occur months or years after a disease is diagnosed or after treatment has ended. Late effects may be caused by cancer or cancer treatment. They may include physical, mental, and social health issues, and second cancers. The sooner late effects are treated the better. Ask your care team about what late effects could occur. This will help you know what to look for.

Survivorship

A person is a cancer survivor from the time of diagnosis until the end of life. After treatment, your health will be monitored for side effects of treatment and the return of cancer. This is part of your survivorship care plan. It is important to keep any follow-up doctor visits and imaging test appointments. Seek good routine medical care, including regular doctor visits for preventive care and cancer screening.

A personalized survivorship care plan will contain a summary of possible long-term effects of treatment called late effects and list follow-up tests. Find out how your primary care provider will coordinate with specialists for your follow-up care. As you age and the longer you are on a TKI, consider incorporating other team members such as cardio-oncologists.

Side effects

Some potential side effects are described next. They are not listed in order of importance. Some side effects are very rare.

It is very important to take care of yourself by eating well, drinking plenty of fluids, exercising, and doing things that make you feel energized.

Anemia, neutropenia, and thrombocytopenia

Some cancer treatments can cause low blood cell counts.

- **Anemia** is a condition where your body does not have enough healthy blood cells, resulting in less oxygen being carried to your cells. You might tire easily if you are anemic.
- **Neutropenia** is a decrease in neutrophils, the most common type of white blood cell. This puts you at risk for infection.
- **Thrombocytopenia** is a condition where there are not enough platelets found in the blood. This puts you at risk for bleeding.

Diarrhea

Diarrhea is frequent and watery bowel movements. Your care team will tell you how to manage diarrhea. It is important to drink lots of fluids.

Distress

Depression, anxiety, and sleeping problems are common and are a normal part of cancer diagnosis. Talk to your care team and with those whom you feel most comfortable about how you are feeling. There are services, people, and medicine that can help you. Support and counseling services are available.

Fatigue

Fatigue is a state of physical or mental tiredness that can be characterized by a lack of energy, motivation, or stamina. Fatigue may be caused by cancer or it may be a side effect of treatment. Let your care team know how you are feeling and if fatigue is getting in the way of doing the things you enjoy. Eating a balanced diet, exercise, yoga, acupuncture, and massage therapy can help. You might be referred to a nutritionist or dietitian to help with fatigue.

Infection

Infections occur more frequently and are more severe in those with a weakened immune system. Drug treatment for CML can weaken the body's natural defense against infections. If not treated early, infections can be fatal.

Neutropenia, a low number of white blood cells, can lead to frequent or severe infections. When someone with neutropenia also develops a fever, it is called febrile neutropenia (FN). With FN, your risk of severe infection may be higher than normal. This is because a low number of white blood cells leads to a reduced ability to fight infections. FN is a side effect of some types of systemic therapy.

Nausea and vomiting

Nausea and vomiting are common side effects of treatment. You will be given medicine to prevent nausea and vomiting.

Neuropathy

Neuropathy is a nerve problem that causes pain, numbness, tingling, swelling, or muscle weakness in different parts of the body. It usually begins in the hands or feet and gets worse over time. Neuropathy may be caused by cancer or cancer treatment.

Neurotoxicity

Some treatments can damage the nervous system (neurotoxicity) causing problems with concentration and memory. Seizures and confusion can occur.

Pain

Tell your care team about any pain or discomfort. You might meet with a palliative care specialist or with a pain specialist to manage pain. Some people may benefit from palliative radiation therapy or ablation therapy to help relieve pain. During this treatment, a radiation beam is focused on the tumor.

Quality of life

Cancer and its treatment can affect your overall well-being or quality of life.

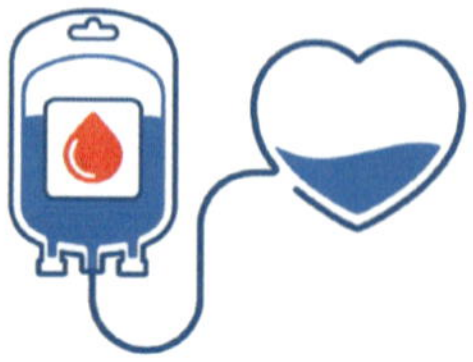

Transfusions

A transfusion is a common procedure to replace blood or blood components (red blood cells or platelets). It is given through an intravenous (IV) line, a tiny tube that is inserted into a vein with a small needle.

- ✓ The whole process can take about 1 to 4 hours, depending on how much blood is needed.
- ✓ Most transfusions use blood from a donor. Some people choose a family member or friend to donate blood.
- ✓ Blood transfusions are usually very safe. Donated blood is carefully tested, handled, and stored.
- ✓ Most people's bodies handle blood transfusions very well. But, like any medical procedure, there are some risks. Speak with your care team for specific information about your risks.
- ✓ Systemic therapy can affect how bone marrow makes new blood cells. Some people getting treatment for cancer might need a transfusion of red blood cells or platelets.

Key points

- CML is usually treated with targeted therapy. Targeted therapy focuses on specific or unique features of cancer cells.
- A tyrosine kinase inhibitor (TKI) is a type of targeted therapy that blocks the signals that cause certain cancers to grow and spread.
- A hematopoietic cell transplant (HCT) replaces damaged bone marrow stem cells with healthy stem cells.
- A clinical trial is a type of medical research study.
- All cancer treatments can cause unwanted health issues called side effects. It is important for you to tell your care team about all your side effects so they can be managed.

Questions to ask

- What phase is my CML and how does the phase affect my treatment options?
- What can I expect from treatment?
- Are there resources to help me pay for treatment or other care I may need?
- Am I candidate for a clinical trial?
- How will you treat side effects?

Supportive care resources

More information on supportive care is available at NCCN.org/patientguidelines and on the NCCN Patient Guides for Cancer app.

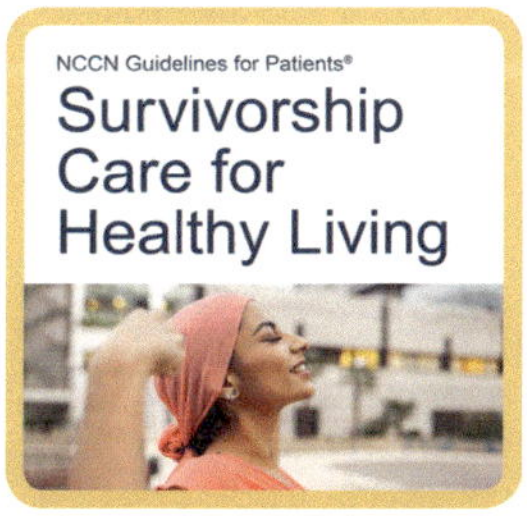

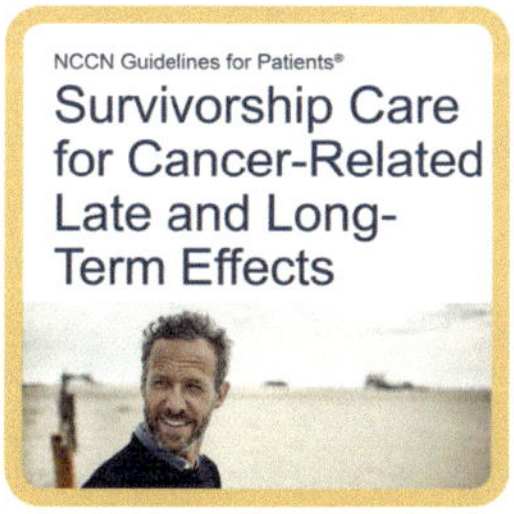

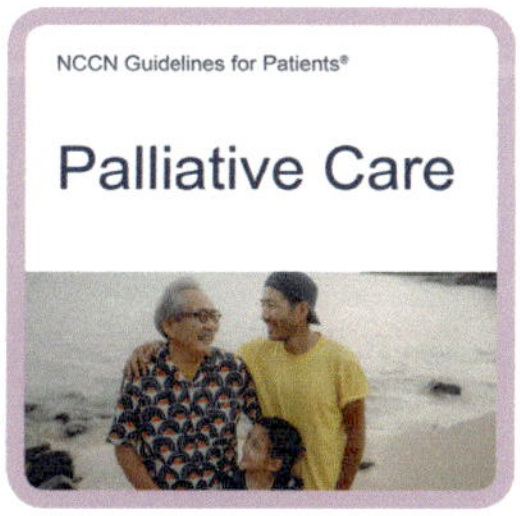

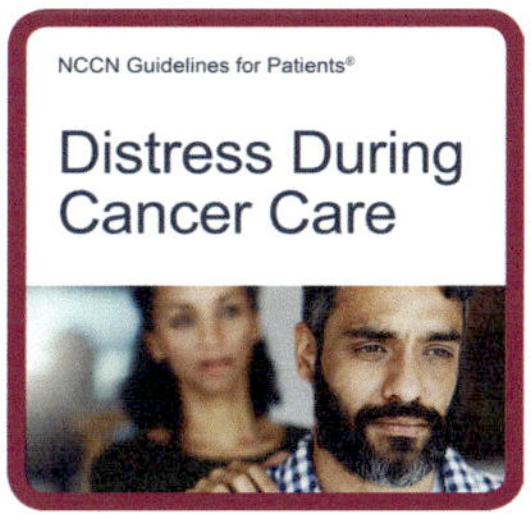

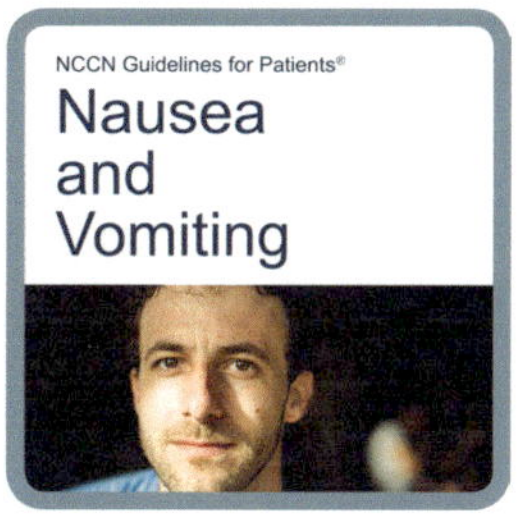

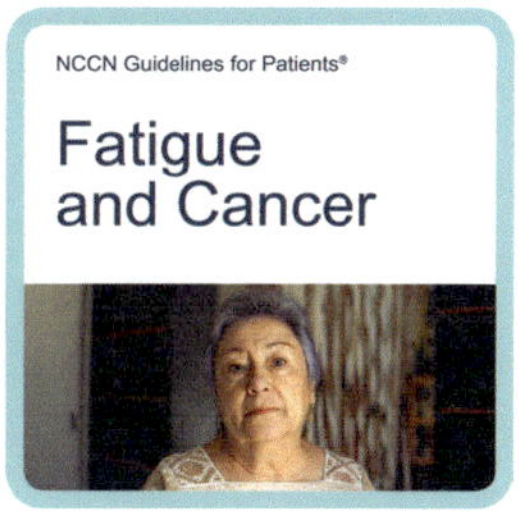

4
Chronic phase

In chronic phase CML (CP-CML), there is an increased number of granulocytes in the blood, bone marrow, or both. CP-CML is treatable. Together, you and your care team will choose a treatment plan that is best for you.

Overview

CML is often diagnosed during the chronic phase of the disease. In this phase, there is an increased number of white blood cells called granulocytes in the blood, bone marrow, or both. Less than 15 out of every 100 blood cells are blasts (<15%) in chronic phase CML (CP-CML).

CP-CML responds well to treatment. However, if left untreated, CP-CML can progress to accelerated phase (AP-CML) or blast phase CML (BP-CML), which is more difficult to cure.

CP-CML is highly treatable. Treatment includes targeted therapy or tyrosine kinase inhibitors (TKIs). Keep up with follow-up visits and testing. You can expect a near-normal to normal life expectancy if CML goes into remission and you continue to take medicine as prescribed.

Not everyone's disease responds to treatment in the same way. Some people will do better than expected. Others will do worse. Factors such as your general health or if you have serious health conditions are also very important.

Guide 2
Risk groups

Low	• Sokal score is less than 0.8 • Hasford (EURO) score is 780 or less • EUTOS long-term survival (ELTS) score is 1.5680 or less
Intermediate	• Sokal score is between 0.8 and 1.2 • Hasford (EURO) score is between 781 and 1480 • EUTOS score is between 1.5680 and 2.2185
High	• Sokal score is more than 1.2 • Hasford (EURO) score is more than 1480 • EUTOS score is more than 2.2185

Risk groups

People in the same risk group will likely respond to treatment in the same way. As a result, doctors often use risk groups to help plan treatment. Ask how your risk group will affect your treatment. **See Guide 2.**

In CML, risk is calculated using:

- Age
- Spleen size on physical exam
- Blood counts

Based on this information, you will receive one of the following:

- Sokal score
- Hasford (EURO) score
- EUTOS long-term survival (ELTS) score

This score places you into a risk group:

- Low
- Intermediate
- High

In addition to your risk score, these factors are important:

- If you have any other serious health issues called comorbidities
- Side effects and toxicity of a tyrosine kinase inhibitor (TKI)
- Possible drug interactions between a chosen TKI and any medicines, herbals, supplements, and over-the-counter (OTC) drugs you are taking
- Whether your insurance plan will cover a particular TKI (there are lower-cost generic TKIs available)
- Your wishes or preferences about treatment options

Primary treatment

The first or main treatment given is called primary treatment. It is based on your risk group.

Low risk

For low risk, the preferred treatment options are:

- Imatinib or generic imatinib (generic imatinib is the same in dosage, safety, strength, quality, and performance as imatinib)
- Second-generation TKI (bosutinib, dasatinib, or nilotinib)
- Clinical trial

Intermediate or high risk

For intermediate or high risk, the preferred treatment option is a second-generation TKI (bosutinib, dasatinib, or nilotinib). Imatinib or generic imatinib and a clinical trial are also options.

Monitoring

To see how well CML is responding to targeted therapy, you will be monitored with qPCR using the International Scale (IS). A qPCR (IS) is the only tool sensitive enough to detect very low levels of *BCR::ABL1*.

qPCR (IS) scores

The qPCR (IS) score uses a standard baseline of 100%. This is the starting point or value that your results are measured against. It is the average of what is observed in untreated individuals; it is possible to have a value of greater than 100%. Changes in qPCR (IS) scores are often described in terms of log changes. Log changes can decrease or increase. A log increase means that the value has gone up at least 10 times from the lowest it has been. For example, an increase of *BCR::ABL1* to 1.2% from a previous value of 0.12% would be a one log increase. A log increase while being treated is cause for concern and would prompt your oncologist to re-evaluate your CML.

Guide 3
Response types and definitions

Complete hematologic (blood) response (CHR)	• Blood counts are normal • No immature cells, such as myelocytes, promyelocytes, or blasts in blood • No signs and symptoms of disease (spleen is normal size)
Cytogenetic (Philadelphia chromosome) response	• Complete cytogenetic response (CCyR): No Philadelphia chromosomes are found (Ph-) • Major cytogenetic response (MCyR): Ph+ are between 0% and 35% • Partial cytogenetic response (PCyR): Ph+ are between 1% and 35% • Minor cytogenetic response: Ph+ are between 36% and 65%
Molecular *(BCR::ABL1)* response	• Early molecular response (EMR): *BCR::ABL1* (IS) is 10% or less at 3 and 6 months • Major molecular response (MMR): *BCR::ABL1* (IS) is 0.1% or less • Deep molecular response (DMR): *BCR::ABL1* (IS) is 0.01% or less (MR4.0) or *BCR::ABL1* (IS) is 0.0032% or less (MR4.5)
Relapse	• Any sign of loss of response

Response milestones

For CML, treatment results are discussed in terms of response milestones. The goal is to reach certain response milestones within a specific timeframe and maintain those milestones.

Some important milestones are as follows:

- **Early molecular response (EMR)** is defined as *BCR::ABL1* less than 10% at 3 months and 6 months. It is a sign of how well treatment will work in the long term. The next milestone is complete cytogenetic response by 12 months.
- **Complete cytogenetic response (CCyR)** is the absence of the Philadelphia chromosome (Ph-). *BCR::ABL1* is 1% or less. A CCyR should be achieved within 12 months.
- **Major molecular response (MMR)** is defined as *BCR::ABL1* less than 0.1%. MMR can predict a deep molecular response.
- **Deep molecular response (DMR)** is when *BCR::ABL1* can't be detected except by the most sensitive of tests, or cannot be detected at all. In a DMR, *BCR::ABL1* (IS) is at 0.01% or less.

For treatment milestones, **see Guide 4.**

Not meeting milestones

If treatment is not meeting certain milestones, then it is possible your CML is resistant to the TKI you are taking.

If this is the case, you will be asked if you:

- Missed or forgot to take any doses
- Are taking any medicines, over-the-counter (OTC) drugs, herbals, or supplements, or if there were any changes to other medicines you might take for your heart, allergies, or digestion.

It is very important to tell your care team about any teas you drink like green tea and any supplements you take such as turmeric. It might be one reason your treatment is not working. Another reason might be that your CML has a new drug-resistant mutation. Your care team will consider this and order any mutation or biomarker testing as needed.

Second-line treatment

Second-line treatment options are based on qPCR (IS) results and if primary treatment milestones were met. Response milestones are measured as the percentage of cells with *BCR::ABL1* using qPCR (IS). The goal is to reduce the number of CML cells with *BCR::ABL1* to less than 1% within 12 months.

Guide 4
Early treatment milestones using *BCR::ABL1 (IS)*

If at 3 months	*BCR::ABL1* (IS) is more than 10%, then possible TKI resistance
	BCR::ABL1 (IS) is between 10% and 1% (EMR), then milestone met
	BCR::ABL1 (IS) is between 1% and 0.1% (CCyR), then milestone met
	BCR::ABL1 (IS) is 0.1% or less (DMR), then milestone met
If at 6 months	*BCR::ABL1* (IS) is more than 10%, then TKI resistance
	BCR::ABL1 (IS) is between 10% and 1% (EMR), then milestone met
	BCR::ABL1 (IS) is between 1% and 0.1% (CCyR), then milestone met
	BCR::ABL1 (IS) is 0.1% or less (DMR), then milestone met
If at 12 months	*BCR::ABL1* (IS) is more than 10%, then TKI resistance
	BCR::ABL1 (IS) is between 10% and 1% (EMR), then possible TKI resistance
	BCR::ABL1 (IS) is between 1% and 0.1% (CCyR), then milestone met if goal is long-term survival. Milestone not met if goal is treatment-free remission.
	BCR::ABL1 (IS) is 0.1% or less (DMR), then milestone met

- Red shows milestone not met.
- Yellow shows area of concern and possible TKI resistance.
- Light green milestone is based on the treatment goal.
- Green shows milestone goal met.
- Orange shows area of concern and possible TKI resistance.

Milestone not met

If the *BCR::ABL1* (IS) level is more than 10% after 6 or more than 1% after 12 months, it means that treatment milestones were not met or maintained. If you have been taking your medicine regularly, the next option is to switch to another TKI (not imatinib) and consider mutation testing. If a hematopoietic cell transplant (HCT) is an option in the future, you might talk with a transplant expert.

Possible TKI resistance

You might have possible TKI resistance if the number of *BCR::ABL1* (IS) cells:

- Is more than 10% after 3 months
- Is more than 1% after 12 months

You might have additional biomarker and mutation testing before continuing treatment. Since a treatment response can still occur with more time, you might remain on the same TKI or switch to a different TKI.

Milestone might have been reached

For those with *BCR::ABL1* (IS) between 0.1% and 1% at 12 months, if the treatment goal is:

- Long-term survival, then the milestone is met and you will continue with the same TKI.
- Treatment-free remission (TFR), then the milestone is not met. You might switch to a different TKI, be referred to a center that specializes in CML, or be recommended for a clinical trial.

Treatment-free remission

For some, it may be possible to discontinue or stop TKI therapy if all milestones have been met. This is called treatment-free remission (TFR). Your care team should consult with a CML specialist and review with you in detail the potential risks and benefits. You will need to agree (consent) to stop therapy and be aware of the TKI withdrawal side effects.

Frequent monitoring is needed for those in remission who have stopped taking TKI therapy. You will need to have blood tests more often. This is to make sure that your *BCR::ABL1* level is closely monitored. If the *BCR::ABL1* level increases above 0.1%, you will need to restart treatment. There is a chance that your cancer might return (relapse) if you stop taking the targeted therapy. Ask your care team about the risks.

Milestone met

If milestones have been reached, you will stay on your TKI. It's very important not to stop your medication without your doctor's advice or skip doses of your medicine. Missing doses allows the leukemia cells to grow and potentially develop TKI resistance. Monitoring will continue indefinitely.

Key points

- In chronic phase CML (CP-CML), there is an increased number of white blood cells called granulocytes found in blood, bone marrow, or both. Less than 15 out of every 100 blood cells are blasts (<15%).
- CP-CML is highly treatable.
- Treatment for CP-CML is based on risk groups using age, spleen size, and blood counts.
- Treatment results are discussed in terms of milestones. The goal is to reach and maintain certain treatment milestones within a specific timeframe.
- Two very important milestones are early molecular response (EMR) at 3 months and 6 months and complete cytogenetic response (CCyR) by 12 months.
- The minimal goal of treatment is to reduce the number of CML cells with *BCR::ABL1* to less than 1% within 12 months.

It is very important to take all medicine exactly as prescribed and not miss or skip doses.

Questions to ask

- What is my risk group and how does this affect my treatment options?
- What are my options if treatment doesn't work as expected?
- What should I do if I miss a dose?
- What decisions must be made today?
- Is there a social worker or someone who can help me decide about treatment?

5
Advanced phase

Accelerated phase (AP) and blast phase (BP) are known as advanced phase CML. These phases are defined by an increase in blasts, additional gene mutations, and leukemia that is spreading. A hematopoietic cell transplant (HCT) would follow blast phase treatment for the best chance of remission. Together, you and your care team will choose a treatment plan that is best for you.

Testing

In accelerated phase CML (AP-CML), the blasts are myeloid. In blast phase CML (BP-CML), the blasts can be myeloid or lymphoid. This is different from chronic phase CML (CP-CML) where all of the blasts are myeloid. Human leukocyte antigen (HLA) testing might be done if a hematopoietic cell transplant (HCT) is planned.

Before treatment, you will have tests to confirm the advanced phase of CML—accelerated or blast phase. The phase is based on the number and type of blasts, if there are any new mutations, and if CML has spread to tissues and organs outside of the bone marrow or blood.

- **In AP-CML and BP-CML**, the percentage of blasts is higher than normal.
- **In BP-CML**, myeloblasts or lymphoblasts may be found in tissues and organs outside the bone marrow or blood. Normal maturation process is impaired.

For definitions of advanced phase CML, **see Guide 5.**

Guide 5
Definitions of advanced phase CML

Accelerated	Any of the following: • Blood myeloblasts are between 15% and 29% • Blood myeloblasts and promyelocytes total 30% or more • Blood basophils are 20% or more • Platelet count is 100 x 10^9/L or less • Additional mutations are found in Ph+ cells • Any increase in lymphoblasts is a concern that blast phase is beginning
Blast	Any of the following: • 30% or more blasts are found in blood, bone marrow, or both • Blast cells are found in tissues and organs outside the bone marrow or blood

Mutation testing

New mutations in the *BCR::ABL1* gene may occur over time. This can happen as CML progresses to advanced phases or it can happen during treatment for CML.

Mutation testing is used to look for these new mutations. Testing can be performed on blood or bone marrow. It should be done prior to starting treatment for advanced phase CML and for any convincing evidence of loss of response to treatment. Some targeted therapies will work on certain mutations, while others will not. Therefore, the tyrosine kinase inhibitor (TKI) chosen will be based on the type of gene mutation(s). Discuss with your care team why a certain treatment is being chosen and how it might work better for your type and phase of CML.

Treatment planning

Factors such as your age, medical history, test results, and any prior TKI therapy will be used for treatment planning. The goal of treatment is to stop CML from progressing to accelerated or blast phase.

Your care team will consider the following when planning treatment for advanced phase CML:

- Did your CML progress while being treated using TKI therapy?
- Did your CML progress while not being treated?
- Are you a candidate for a hematopoietic cell transplant (HCT)?
- Is there any leukemia in your central nervous system (CNS)?
- What mutations does your CML have?
- What TKIs did you take before? Did your CML not respond or was it resistant to certain TKIs?

Accelerated phase

In accelerated phase CML (AP-CML), the percentage of myeloblasts is high. Platelet count might be low. In all phases, CML cells contain the Philadelphia (Ph) chromosome. However, in the accelerated and blast phases, there may be new abnormal changes within chromosomes.

Treatment options

The treatment goal is to stop CML from progressing to blast phase. For long-term control, an allogeneic (donor) HCT is likely needed. For treatment options, **see Guide 6.**

Guide 6 Treatment options: Accelerated phase
Clinical trial
Preferred TKIs • Bosutinib • Dasatinib • Nilotinib • Ponatinib
Used in some cases • Imatinib or generic imatinib • Asciminib

Blast phase

The blasts in blast phase CML (BP-CML) can be myeloid (myeloblasts) or lymphoid (lymphoblasts).

- **In myeloid blast phase**, at least 30 out of every 100 cells (30%) are blasts.
- **In lymphoid blast phase**, any number of abnormal lymphoblasts is concerning.

Blasts may be found in tissues and organs outside the bone marrow or blood. A lumbar puncture might be done if CML is suspected in the fluid that surrounds the spine or brain.

An allogeneic (donor) HCT or intensive chemotherapy would follow initial TKI treatment for blast phase CML.

Blood cell formation

All blood cells start as blood stem cells. A blood stem cell has to go through many stages to become a red blood cell, white blood cell, or platelet. CML affects the myeloid progenitor cells and causes too many granulocytes (a type of white blood cell). However, advanced phase CML can affect the lymphoid progenitor cells.

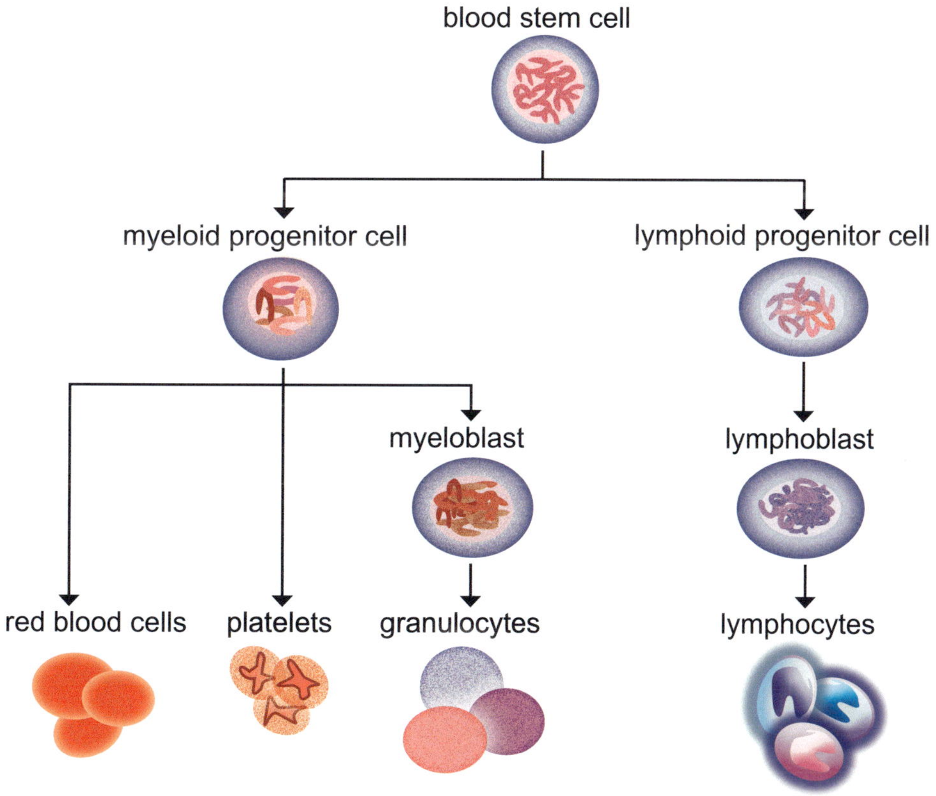

Treatment options

Options for lymphoid blast phase include:

- Clinical trial
- Acute lymphoblastic leukemia (ALL)-type induction chemotherapy with a TKI (preferred)
- TKI with steroids

More information on ALL-type induction therapies is available at NCCN.org/patientguidelines and on the NCCN Patient Guides for Cancer app.

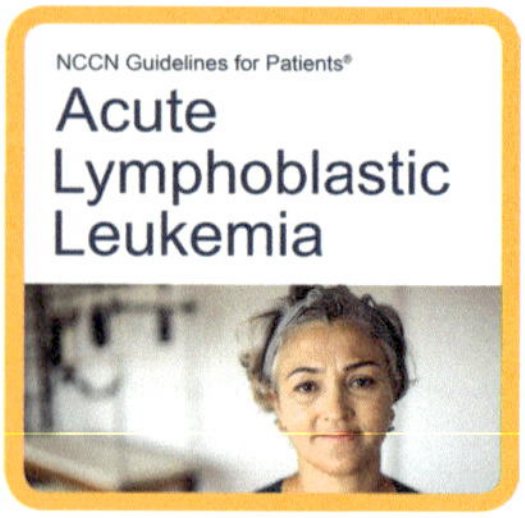

Options for myeloid blast phase include:

- Clinical trial
- Acute myeloid leukemia (AML)-type induction chemotherapy with a TKI (preferred)
- TKI

More information on AML-type induction therapies is available at NCCN.org/patientguidelines and on the NCCN Patient Guides for Cancer app.

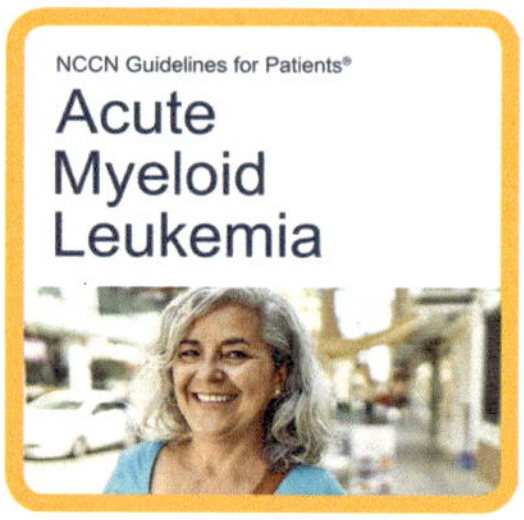

After an HCT

A hematopoietic cell transplant (HCT) is used to prevent CML from progressing. It is a treatment given to cure CML. However, this does not always happen. An allogeneic HCT uses healthy blood (hematopoietic) stem cells from a donor who may or may not be related to you.

How your body responds to an HCT is based on age, if you have other serious health issues (comorbidities), donor type, and transplant center. You will have qPCR (IS) after an HCT to see if any cells with the Philadelphia chromosome or *BCR::ABL1* gene remain.

In a complete cytogenetic response (CCyR), no Philadelphia chromosomes remain and *BCR::ABL1* level is 1% or less.

CCyR

Following an HCT, you will be monitored with qPCR. This is done with blood, and/or bone marrow. qPCR will be done every 3 months for 2 years, then every 3 to 6 months. If qPCR is negative, then you will continue to be monitored. You might have TKI therapy for at least one year after transplant if you had accelerated phase CML (AP-CML) or blast phase CML (BP-CML) before.

Not in CCyR or in relapse

If Philadelphia chromosomes or *BCR::ABL1* genes remain after the HCT, or CML has returned, then treatment options include:

- TKI
- TKI with donor lymphocyte infusion (DLI)
- Clinical trial

In a DLI you will receive white blood cells from the same person who donated blood-forming cells for the HCT. Treatment options are based on the type(s) of TKI you had before, your current health, *BCR::ABL1* mutations, and other factors. Your wishes are also important.

In a complete cytogenetic response (CCyR), no Philadelphia chromosomes remain.

Key points

- Accelerated phase and blast phase are known as advanced phase CML. These phases are defined by an increase in blasts, additional gene mutations, and leukemia that is spreading.
- In all phases, CML cells contain the Philadelphia (Ph) chromosome. However, in the accelerated phase, there may be new abnormal changes within chromosomes (gene mutations).
- TKIs are often used to treat advanced phase CML. Chemotherapy or steroids may be added if in blast phase. For long-term control, an allogeneic (donor) hematopoietic cell transplant (HCT) is needed.

Questions to ask

- Which treatment do you recommend and why?
- Does this treatment offer a cure? If not, how well can treatment stop the cancer from growing?
- Does the order of treatment matter?
- What side effects can I expect from this treatment?
- Am I candidate for an allogeneic HCT?

6
Other resources

Want to learn more? Here's how you can get additional help.

What else to know

This book can help you improve your cancer care. It plainly explains expert recommendations and suggests questions to ask your care team. But, it's not the only resource that you have.

You're welcome to receive as much information and help as you need. Many people are interested in learning more about:

- The details of their health and treatment
- Being a part of a care team
- Getting financial help
- Finding a care provider who is an expert in their field
- Coping with side effects

What else to do

Your health care center can help you with next steps. They often have on-site resources to help meet your needs and find answers to your questions. Health care centers can also inform you of resources in your community.

In addition to help from your providers, the resources listed in the next section provide support for many people like yourself. Look through the list and visit the provided websites to learn more about these organizations

Where to get help

AnCan Foundation
ancan.org

BMT InfoNet (Blood & Marrow Transplant Information Network)
BMTInfoNet.org

Cancer*Care*
Cancercare.org

Cancer Hope Network
cancerhopenetwork.org

Imerman Angels
Imermanangels.org

Leukemia Research Foundation
leukemiarf.org

MedlinePlus
medlineplus.gov

National Bone Marrow Transplant Link (nbmtLINK)
nbmtLINK.org

National Cancer Institute (NCI)
cancer.gov/types/leukemia

National Coalition for Cancer Survivorship
canceradvocacy.org

NMDP
nmdp.org

The Leukemia & Lymphoma Society (LLS)
LLS.org/PatientSupport

Triage Cancer
triagecancer.org

Questions to ask

- Who can I talk to about help with housing, food, and other basic needs?
- What help is available for transportation, childcare, and home care?
- What other services are available to me and my caregivers?
- How can I connect with others and build a support system?
- Who can I talk to if I don't feel safe at home, at work, or in my neighborhood?

Finding a clinical trial

In the United States

NCCN Cancer Centers
NCCN.org/cancercenters

The National Cancer Institute (NCI)
cancer.gov/about-cancer/treatment/clinical-trials/search

Worldwide

The U.S. National Library of Medicine (NLM)
clinicaltrials.gov

Need help finding a clinical trial?

NCI's Cancer Information Service (CIS)
1.800.4.CANCER (1.800.422.6237)
cancer.gov/contact

Words to know

accelerated phase CML (AP-CML)
The second phase of chronic myeloid leukemia progression, when the number of blast cells is increased.

acute lymphoblastic leukemia (ALL)
A fast-growing cancer that causes too many immature white blood cells called lymphoblasts to be made.

acute myeloid leukemia (AML)
A fast-growing cancer that causes too many immature white blood cells called myeloblasts to be made.

advanced phase
A rating of chronic myeloid leukemia, when the number of immature blood cells (blast cells) is high and it is causing symptoms.

allogeneic hematopoietic cell transplant (HCT)
A treatment in which the patient receives healthy, immature blood-forming cells from another person to replace damaged or diseased cells in the bone marrow. Also called allogeneic stem cell transplant (SCT).

***BCR::ABL1* gene**
An abnormal gene that is formed when the *BCR* gene and *ABL1* gene join on the Philadelphia chromosome. Also called *BCR::ABL1* fusion gene.

BCR::ABL1 protein
An abnormal protein that is made by the *BCR::ABL1* fusion gene and causes too many abnormal white blood cells to be made.

blast cell
An immature white blood cell. Can be myeloid or lymphoid.

blast phase CML (BP-CML)
The final phase of chronic myeloid leukemia, which has the highest number of blast cells in the blood and bone marrow and can be life-threatening. Blasts can be myeloid or lymphoid. Also called blast crisis.

blood stem cell
An immature blood-forming cell from which all other types of blood cells are made. Also called hematopoietic stem cell.

bone marrow
The soft, sponge-like tissue in the center of most bones where blood cells are made.

bone marrow aspiration
The removal of a small amount of liquid bone marrow to test for disease.

bone marrow biopsy
The removal of a small amount of solid bone and bone marrow to test for disease.

chemotherapy
Drugs that kill fast-dividing cells, including cancer cells and normal cells.

chromosomes
Long strands that contain bundles of coded instructions (genes) in cells for making and controlling cells.

chronic myeloid leukemia (CML)
A slow-growing cancer that starts in the bone marrow and causes too many granulocytes to form.

chronic phase CML (CP-CML)
The first phase of chronic myeloid leukemia, when the number of white blood cells is higher than normal but may not cause symptoms.

complete cytogenetic response (CCyR)
When tests don't find any copies of the Philadelphia chromosome.

cytogenetics
The study of chromosomes.

deep molecular response (DMR)
No copies of the abnormal *BCR::ABL1* gene or copies are detected at a very low level using a very sensitive test.

donor lymphocyte infusion (DLI)
Procedure in which a person receives white blood cells from the same person who donated blood-forming cells for the hematopoietic cell transplant.

early molecular response (EMR)
When *BCR::ABL1* is less than 10% at 3 months and 6 months.

flow cytometry
A test that looks at certain substances on the surface of cells to identify the type of cells present.

fluorescence in situ hybridization (FISH)
A lab test that uses special dyes to look for abnormal changes in a cell's genes.

fusion gene
A gene that is made when parts of two separate genes join.

gene
A set of coded instructions in cells for making new cells and controlling how cells behave.

graft-versus-host disease (GVHD)
A disease that occurs when transplanted blood stem cells attack a patient's normal cells.

granulocyte
A type of white blood cell that has small particles (granules).

hematologist
A doctor who's an expert in diseases of the blood.

hematopathologist
A doctor who specializes in blood diseases by looking at cells under a microscope.

hematopoietic cell
An immature blood-forming cell from which all other types of blood cells are made. Also called blood stem cell.

hematopoietic cell transplant (HCT)
A treatment that replaces damaged or diseased cells in the bone marrow with healthy blood-forming cells. Also called stem cell transplant (SCT) or bone marrow transplant (BMT).

human leukocyte antigen (HLA)
Special proteins on the surface of cells that help the body to tell its own cells apart from foreign cells.

immune system
The body's natural defense against infection and disease.

International Scale (IS)
A standardized scale for measuring and reporting results of a very sensitive test that measures the number of cells that have the *BCR::ABL1* gene.

log reduction
A decrease in the number of cells that have the *BCR::ABL1* gene.

lymphoid
Referring to a type of white blood cell called a lymphocyte.

major molecular response (MMR)
An improvement related to treatment, when tests detect a 3-log reduction in *BCR::ABL1* levels. It means that there are 1,000 times

fewer cells with the *BCR::ABL1* gene than the standardized baseline level.

molecular response
An improvement related to treatment, when tests detect a decrease in the number of cells that have the *BCR::ABL1* gene.

mutation testing
A test that looks for abnormal changes in genes (the coded instructions in cells for making and controlling cells).

myeloid
Referring to a type of white blood cell called a granulocyte.

pathologist
A doctor who's an expert in testing cells and tissue to find disease.

Philadelphia (Ph) chromosome
An abnormal, short chromosome 22 that is formed when parts of chromosomes 9 and 22 switch with each other. It is the hallmark of chronic myeloid leukemia and contains the *BCR::ABL1* gene.

prognosis
The likely or expected course and outcome of a disease.

quantitative reverse transcriptase polymerase chain reaction (qPCR)
A very sensitive test that measures the number of cells in the blood or bone marrow that have the *BCR::ABL1* gene.

relapse
The return or worsening of cancer after a period of improvement.

remission
There are minor or no signs of a disease.

resistance
When cancer does not respond to a drug treatment.

second-line treatment
The next treatment used against a disease after the first treatment failed or had to be stopped.

supportive care
Treatment for the symptoms or health conditions caused by cancer or cancer treatment.

targeted therapy
Treatment with drugs that target a specific or unique feature of cancer cells.

transfusion
Replacing lost blood with new blood.

translocation
When pieces of two chromosomes (long strands of coded instructions for controlling cells) break off and switch with each other.

treatment response
An outcome or improvement in disease that is caused by treatment.

tyrosine kinase inhibitor (TKI)
A type of drug that attaches to the BCR::ABL1 protein so that it can't send growth signals.

NCCN Contributors

This patient guide is based on the NCCN Clinical Practice Guidelines in Oncology (NCCN Guidelines®) for Chronic Myeloid Leukemia, Version 1.2025. It was adapted, reviewed, and published with help from the following people:

Dorothy A. Shead, MS
Senior Director
Patient Information Operations

Tanya Fischer, MEd, MSLIS
Senior Medical Writer

Susan Kidney
Senior Graphic Design Specialist

The NCCN Clinical Practice Guidelines in Oncology (NCCN Guidelines®) for Chronic Myeloid Leukemia, Version 1.2025 were developed by the following NCCN Panel Members:

*Neil P. Shah, MD, PhD/Chair
UCSF Helen Diller Family Comprehensive Cancer Center

*Ravi Bhatia, MD/Vice-Chair
O'Neal Comprehensive Cancer Center at UAB

Jessica K. Altman, MD
Robert H. Lurie Comprehensive Cancer Center of Northwestern University

Maria Amaya, MD, PhD
University of Colorado Cancer Center

Kebede H. Begna, MD
Mayo Clinic Comprehensive Cancer Center

Ellin Berman, MD
Memorial Sloan Kettering Cancer Center

Onyee Chan, MD
Moffitt Cancer Center

*Joan Clements
CML Buster Foundation

Robert H. Collins, Jr., MD
UT Southwestern Simmons Comprehensive Cancer Center

Peter T. Curtin, MD
City of Hope National Medical Center

Daniel J. DeAngelo, MD, PhD
Dana-Farber/Brigham and Women's Cancer Center

Michael Drazer, MD, PhD
The UChicago Medicine Comprehensive Cancer Center

Lori Maness, MD
Fred and Pamela Buffett Cancer Center

Leland Metheny, MD
Case Comprehensive Cancer Center/ University Hospitals Seidman Cancer Center and Cleveland Clinic Taussig Cancer Institute

Sanjay Mohan, MD, MSCI
Vanderbilt-Ingram Cancer Center

Vivian Oehler, MD
Fred Hutchinson Cancer Center

Iskra Pusic, MD, MSCI
Siteman Cancer Center at Barnes-Jewish Hospital and Washington University School of Medicine

*Lindsay Rein, MD
Duke Cancer Institute

Michal G. Rose, MD
Yale Cancer Center/Smilow Cancer Hospital

Koji Sasaki, MD, PhD
The University of Texas MD Anderson Cancer Center

*William Shomali, MD
Stanford Cancer Institute

B. Douglas Smith, MD
Johns Hopkins Kimmel Cancer Center

*Michael Styler, MD
Fox Chase Cancer Center

Moshe Talpaz, MD
University of Michigan Rogel Cancer Center

Tiffany N. Tanaka, MD
UC San Diego Moores Cancer Center

*Srinivas Tantravahi, MBBS
Huntsman Cancer Institute at the University of Utah

James Thompson, MD, MS
Roswell Park Comprehensive Cancer Center

*Steven Tsai, MD, PhD
UCLA Jonsson Comprehensive Cancer Center

Jennifer Vaughn, MD, MSPH
The Ohio State University Comprehensive Cancer Center - James Cancer Hospital and Solove Research Institute

Jeanna Welborn, MD
UC Davis Comprehensive Cancer Center

*David T. Yang, MD
University of Wisconsin Carbone Cancer Center

NCCN

Kris Gregory, RN, MSN
Senior Vice President, Clinical Information Programs

Hema Sundar, PhD
Senior Manager, Global Clinical Content

* Reviewed this patient guide. For disclosures, visit NCCN.org/disclosures.

NCCN Cancer Centers

Abramson Cancer Center
at the University of Pennsylvania
Philadelphia, Pennsylvania
800.789.7366 • *pennmedicine.org/cancer*

Case Comprehensive Cancer Center/
University Hospitals Seidman Cancer Center and
Cleveland Clinic Taussig Cancer Institute
Cleveland, Ohio
UH Seidman Cancer Center
800.641.2422 • *uhhospitals.org/services/cancer-services*
CC Taussig Cancer Institute
866.223.8100 • *my.clevelandclinic.org/departments/cancer*
Case CCC
216.844.8797 • *case.edu/cancer*

City of Hope National Medical Center
Duarte, California
800.826.4673 • *cityofhope.org*

Dana-Farber/Brigham and Women's Cancer Center |
Mass General Cancer Center
Boston, Massachusetts
877.442.3324 • *youhaveus.org*
617.726.5130 • *massgeneral.org/cancer-center*

Duke Cancer Institute
Durham, North Carolina
888.275.3853 • *dukecancerinstitute.org*

Fox Chase Cancer Center
Philadelphia, Pennsylvania
888.369.2427 • *foxchase.org*

Fred & Pamela Buffett Cancer Center
Omaha, Nebraska
402.559.5600 • *unmc.edu/cancercenter*

Fred Hutchinson Cancer Center
Seattle, Washington
206.667.5000 • *fredhutch.org*

Huntsman Cancer Institute at the University of Utah
Salt Lake City, Utah
800.824.2073 • *healthcare.utah.edu/huntsmancancerinstitute*

Indiana University Melvin and Bren Simon
Comprehensive Cancer Center
Indianapolis, Indiana
888.600.4822 • *www.cancer.iu.edu*

Johns Hopkins Kimmel Cancer Center
Baltimore, Maryland
410.955.8964
www.hopkinskimmelcancercenter.org

Mayo Clinic Comprehensive Cancer Center
Phoenix/Scottsdale, Arizona
Jacksonville, Florida
Rochester, Minnesota
480.301.8000 • Arizona
904.953.0853 • Florida
507.538.3270 • Minnesota
mayoclinic.org/cancercenter

Memorial Sloan Kettering Cancer Center
New York, New York
800.525.2225 • *mskcc.org*

Moffitt Cancer Center
Tampa, Florida
888.663.3488 • *moffitt.org*

O'Neal Comprehensive Cancer Center at UAB
Birmingham, Alabama
800.822.0933 • *uab.edu/onealcancercenter*

Robert H. Lurie Comprehensive Cancer Center
of Northwestern University
Chicago, Illinois
866.587.4322 • *cancer.northwestern.edu*

Roswell Park Comprehensive Cancer Center
Buffalo, New York
877.275.7724 • *roswellpark.org*

Siteman Cancer Center at Barnes-Jewish Hospital
and Washington University School of Medicine
St. Louis, Missouri
800.600.3606 • *siteman.wustl.edu*

St. Jude Children's Research Hospital/
The University of Tennessee Health Science Center
Memphis, Tennessee
866.278.5833 • *stjude.org*
901.448.5500 • *uthsc.edu*

Stanford Cancer Institute
Stanford, California
877.668.7535 • *cancer.stanford.edu*

The Ohio State University Comprehensive Cancer Center
- James Cancer Hospital and Solove Research Institute
Columbus, Ohio
800.293.5066 • *cancer.osu.edu*

The UChicago Medicine Comprehensive Cancer Center
Chicago, Illinois
773.702.1000 • *uchicagomedicine.org/cancer*

The University of Texas MD Anderson Cancer Center
Houston, Texas
844.269.5922 • *mdanderson.org*

UC Davis Comprehensive Cancer Center
Sacramento, California
916.734.5959 • 800.770.9261
health.ucdavis.edu/cancer

UC San Diego Moores Cancer Center
La Jolla, California
858.822.6100 • cancer.ucsd.edu

UCLA Jonsson Comprehensive Cancer Center
Los Angeles, California
310.825.5268 • uclahealth.org/cancer

UCSF Helen Diller Family
Comprehensive Cancer Center
San Francisco, California
800.689.8273 • cancer.ucsf.edu

University of Colorado Cancer Center
Aurora, Colorado
720.848.0300 • coloradocancercenter.org

University of Michigan Rogel Cancer Center
Ann Arbor, Michigan
800.865.1125 • rogelcancercenter.org

University of Wisconsin Carbone Cancer Center
Madison, Wisconsin
608.265.1700 • uwhealth.org/cancer

UT Southwestern Simmons
Comprehensive Cancer Center
Dallas, Texas
214.648.3111 • utsouthwestern.edu/simmons

Vanderbilt-Ingram Cancer Center
Nashville, Tennessee
877.936.8422 • vicc.org

Yale Cancer Center/Smilow Cancer Hospital
New Haven, Connecticut
855.4.SMILOW • yalecancercenter.org

share with us.

Take our survey and help make the NCCN Guidelines for Patients better for everyone!

NCCN.org/patients/comments

Index

Made in United States
Cleveland, OH
07 January 2025

13200817R00036